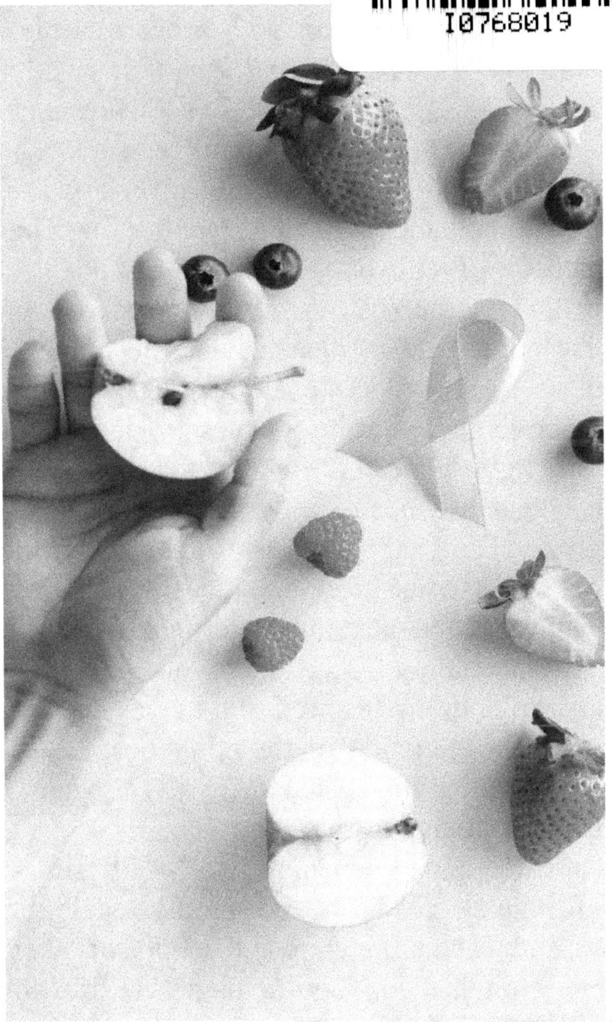

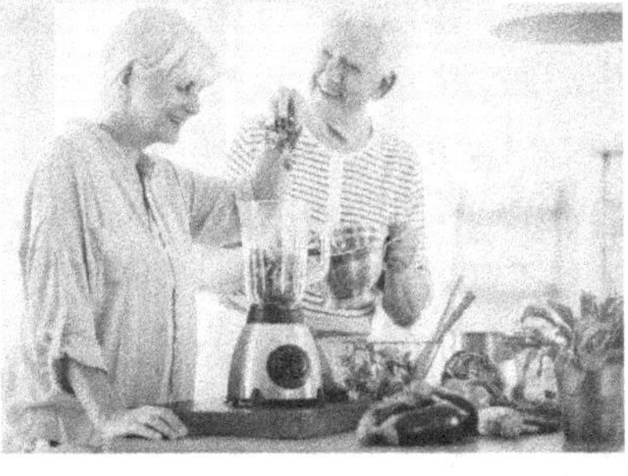

INTRODUCTION

Kingston, a retired librarian with a heart as big as the books on his beloved library's shelves, lived in the peaceful village of Willowbrook, surrounded by towering oak trees and meandering streams. Kingston eventually faced an unexpected adversary: Type 2 diabetes, The diagnosis placed a pall over Kingston's once exuberant life, leaving him with a sudden sense of fragility and insecurity. As he navigated the maze of food restrictions and medical advice, he found himself adrift in a sea of bewilderment and anxiety, longing for a ray of hope to guide him to wellness. Amidst the chaos, a ray of light appeared in the form of a tattered cookbook that had been gathering dust on the shelf of his kitchen: "The Diabetes Diet Cookbook for Seniors." The cookbook, with its tattered cover and dog-eared pages, appealed to Kingston, offering a lifeline in the middle of uncertainty. Kingston set out on a journey of culinary exploration, inspired by the ageless wisdom weaved within the pages of the cookbook. Each recipe became a tribute to his unshakable will to regain control of his health and vigour.

Kingston entered his kitchen, armed with fresh food and a hopeful heart, ready to go on a transformational journey. With each knife chop and spoon stir, he brought the recipes on the cookbook's pages to life, imbuing them with a sense of purpose and passion that matched the depths of his own spirit. Kingston found refuge in the kitchen's warm embrace, amongst the maelstrom of emotions that had enveloped him. The repetitive cadence of slicing vegetables, as well as the delicious perfume of herbs and spices, became his retreat, a haven from the storm of uncertainty that raged beyond his door. Kingston discovered a newfound sense of

THE COMPREHENSIVE DIABETES DIET COOKBOOK FOR SENIORS

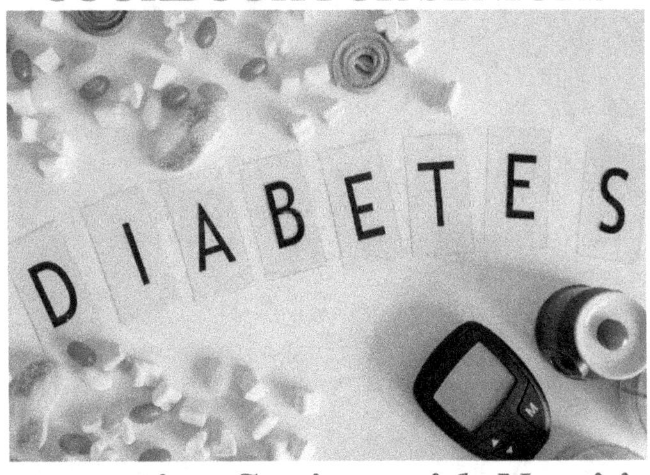

Empowering Seniors with Nutritious Choices for Diabetes Management

Paula C. Brann

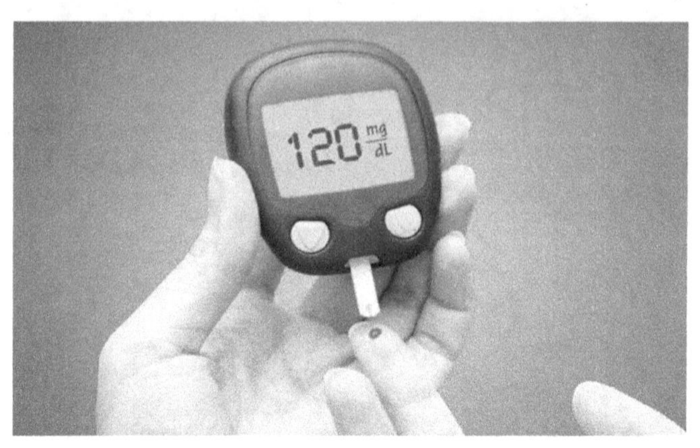

Table of Contents

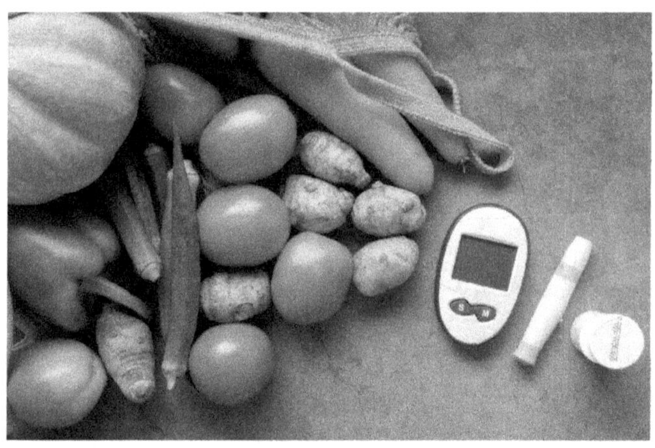

creativity and inventiveness, which ignited a spark of inspiration within him. He experimented with bold flavours and nutritious ingredients, transforming everyday vegetables and lean proteins into gourmet masterpieces that danced on the tongue.

Kingston's journey was far from ended. Armed with newfound understanding and unshakeable faith, he welcomed each new day with a sense of purpose and thankfulness, savouring the little pleasures that lined his path. And as he closed the aged pages of the cookbook, he saw that the most important recipe of all was written within the depths of his own heart. With each meal, Kingston developed a stronger connection to the rich tapestry of flavours on his plate, savouring each mouthful with reverence and appreciation. The once-dreadful spectre of diabetes began to fade, replaced with a sense of empowerment and resilience that penetrated every facet of his personality. Beyond the limits of his kitchen, Kingston's path acted as a beacon of hope for those around him, inspiring those who faced similar hardshipsHis unshakable resolve and indomitable spirit became a symbol of the transformational power of tenacity and resilience, as well as the limitless potential that each of us possesses.

As the sun set below the horizon, leaving a golden colour on the landscape, Kingston sat at his kitchen table, a sense of calm sweeping over him like a soft tide. In the pages of the diabetes diet cookbook, he discovered not just recipes but also a path to wellness, a monument to the human spirit's endurance and the transformational power of food.

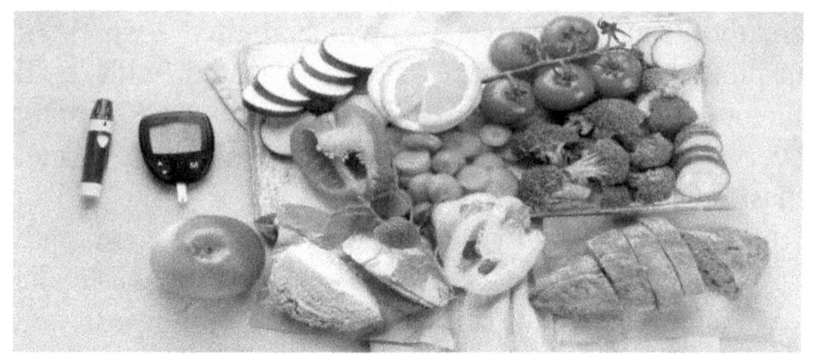

CHAPTER 1: BREAKFAST RECIPES

Oatmeal with Berries and Nuts

Ingredients:
- 1/2 cup old-fashioned rolled oats
- 1 cup water
- 1/4 teaspoon ground cinnamon
- 1/4 cup mixed berries (such as blueberries, strawberries, raspberries)
- 2 tablespoons chopped nuts (such as walnuts, almonds, or pecans)
- 1 teaspoon chia seeds (optional)
- 1/2 teaspoon vanilla extract (optional)
- 1 teaspoon honey or maple syrup (optional, for sweetness)

Instructions :
1. In a small saucepan, bring water to a boil over medium heat.
2. Stir in the rolled oats and decrease the heat to low. Cook the oats, stirring regularly, for 5-7

minutes, or until they reach the desired consistency. Add more water if necessary.

3. When the oats are done, remove the saucepan from the heat. For added flavour, stir in the ground cinnamon and, if using, the vanilla extract.
4. Transfer cooked muesli to a serving bowl.
5. Top the muesli with mixed berries and chopped nuts.
6. If desired, sprinkle chia seeds over the muesli to increase the fibre and omega-3 fatty acid content.
7. If you want to make the muesli sweeter, drizzle it with a teaspoon of honey or maple syrup. Note: If you're watching your sugar intake, avoid adding sweeteners.
8. Serve warm and enjoy a nutritious breakfast to start the day off right!

Greek Yogurt Parfait

Ingredients :
- 1/2 cup of plain, non-fat Greek yogurt
- 1/4 cup of fresh blueberries
- 1/4 cup of fresh strawberries, sliced
- 1 tablespoon of chopped nuts (such as almonds or walnuts)
- 1 teaspoon of ground flaxseeds
- 1/2 teaspoon of cinnamon
- 1 teaspoon of honey (optional, adjust according to dietary needs)
- Fresh mint leaves for garnish (optional)

Instructions :

1. Prepare Ingredients: Wash and slice the strawberries. Measure the blueberries, nuts, and ground flaxseed.
2. Layer Yoghurt: In a glass or dish, begin by stacking half of the Greek yoghurt on the bottom.
3. Add berries: Add half of the blueberries and half of the cut strawberries to the yoghurt.
4. Add nuts and flaxseeds. Sprinkle the berries with half the chopped almonds and half the ground flaxseeds.
5. Repeat Layers: Add the remaining Greek yoghurt, then the remaining berries, almonds, and ground flaxseeds.
6. Sprinkle Cinnamon: Evenly distribute cinnamon over the top of the parfait.
7. Drizzle Honey (Optional): Drizzle a spoonful of honey over the top for extra sweetness. Adjust the amount based on your personal dietary requirements.
8. Garnish:Garnish the parfait with fresh mint leaves for an added punch of flavour and presentation.
9. Serve immediately as a tasty and nutritious breakfast, snack, or dessert for seniors on a diabetes-friendly diet.

Vegetable Egg Muffins

Ingredients :
- 6 large eggs
- 1/4 cup low-fat milk or unsweetened almond milk
- 1/2 cup diced bell peppers (red, green, yellow)
- 1/2 cup diced tomatoes
- 1/2 cup diced onions

- 1/2 cup chopped spinach leaves
- 1/4 cup shredded low-fat cheese (cheddar, mozzarella, or your choice)
- Salt and pepper to taste
- Cooking spray or olive oil for greasing muffin tin

Instructions :

1. Preheat the oven to 350°F (175° C). To prevent sticking, grease a muffin tray with cooking spray or olive oil.
2. In a mixing dish, crack the eggs and lightly beat using a whisk or fork. Add the milk and stir until thoroughly mixed.
3. Combine the chopped spinach, diced bell peppers, onions, tomatoes, and mushrooms with the egg mixture. Season with salt and pepper to taste.
4. Pour the egg and veggie mixture evenly into the prepared muffin cups, filling them about 3/4 full.
5. Bake in the preheated oven for 20-25 minutes, or until the egg muffins are firm and faintly brown on top. To test for doneness, poke a toothpick into the centre of the muffin; if it comes out clean, they're ready.
6. Once completed, remove the muffin tray from the oven and allow the egg muffins to cool for a few minutes before carefully removing them from the tin.
7. Serve the vegetable egg muffins warm or room temperature. These muffins can be refrigerated in an airtight container for 3-4 days. They can also be stored for later use; simply thaw overnight in the fridge and reheat in the microwave or oven before serving.

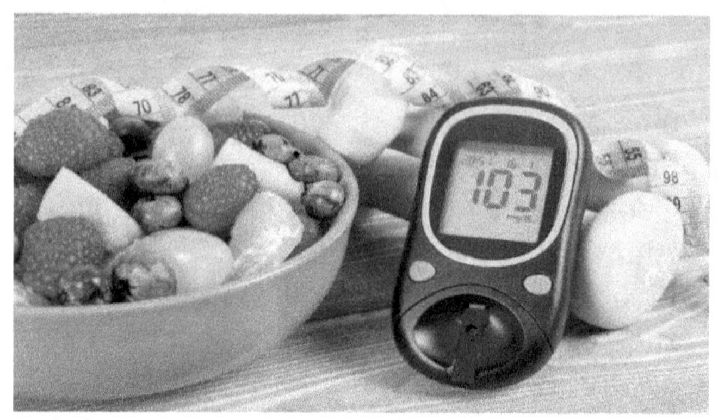

Avocado Toast with Poached Egg

Ingredients :
- 1 ripe avocado
- 2 slices of whole grain bread (low-sodium, if available)
- 2 large eggs
- Salt and pepper to taste
- Optional toppings: sliced tomatoes, baby spinach leaves, crushed red pepper flakes

Instructions :
1. To prepare the Avocado Spread:
2. Cut the avocado in half and remove the pit.
3. Place the avocado flesh in a bowl and mash with a fork until smooth.
4. Season the mashed avocado with salt and pepper, to taste. Set aside.
5. Toast the bread:
6. slices till golden brown and crispy.
7. Poach the eggs.

8. Fill a saucepan with water and bring to a moderate simmer on medium heat.
9. Crack an egg into a small bowl or cup.
10. Carefully place the egg in the simmering water. Repeat for the second egg.
11. Poach the eggs for 3-4 minutes, or until the whites are firm but the yolks remain runny.
12. Take the poached eggs out of the water using To drain extra water, use a slotted spoon and set it on a paper towel.
13. For Avocado Toast, spread a liberal layer of mashed avocado on each slice of toasted bread.
14. Place one poached egg on top of each avocado-covered bread.
15. Season with more salt and pepper if required.
16. Garnish with sliced tomatoes, baby spinach leaves, or crushed red pepper flakes for more flavour and nutrition.
17. Serve and enjoy.
18. Serve the Avocado Toast with Poached Egg immediately while still warm.
19. For a well-balanced supper, serve with some fresh fruit or a small salad.

Cottage Cheese Pancakes

Ingredients :
- 1 cup low-fat cottage cheese
- 3 large eggs
- 1/4 cup whole wheat flour or oat flour
- 1 tablespoon unsweetened almond milk or skim milk
- 1 teaspoon vanilla extract

- 1/2 teaspoon ground cinnamon
- Cooking spray or olive oil for cooking

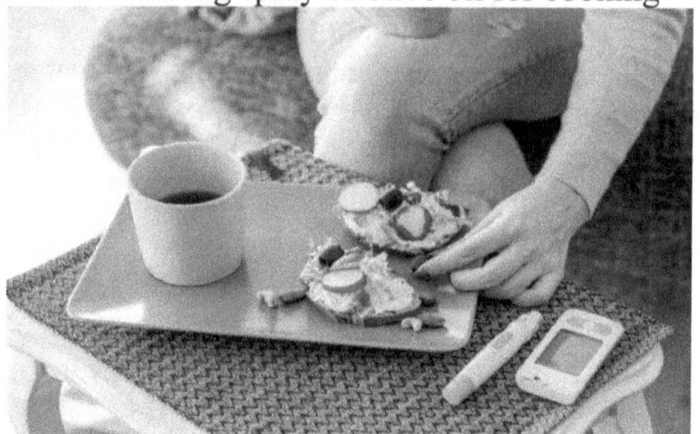

Instructions :

1. In a blender or food processor, combine low-fat cottage cheese, eggs, whole wheat flour, almond milk, vanilla essence, and ground cinnamon. Blend until smooth and thoroughly incorporated.

2. Cook on a nonstick skillet or griddle over medium heat. Coat lightly with cooking spray or a little bit of olive oil.

3. Pour roughly 1/4 cup pancake batter into the skillet for each pancake. Cook until bubbles develop on the pancake's surface and the edges seem firm, which should take about 2-3 minutes.

4. Flip the pancakes and heat for another 1-2 minutes, or until golden brown and fully done.

5. Repeat with the remaining batter, adding additional frying spray or oil to the skillet as needed.

6. Serve the cottage cheese pancakes warm and topped with fresh berries. If preferred, sprinkle with cinnamon or add a dollop of Greek yoghurt.

Smoothie Bowl

Ingredients :
- 1/2 cup frozen berries (such as strawberries, blueberries, or raspberries)
- 1/2 small ripe banana, frozen
- 1/4 cup plain Greek yogurt (low-fat or non-fat)
- 1/4 cup unsweetened almond milk or skim milk
- 1 tablespoon chia seeds or ground flaxseed
- 1/4 teaspoon cinnamon (optional)
- 1/4 cup spinach leaves (optional, for added nutrients)
- Toppings: Sliced fresh fruits (e.g., banana, berries), nuts (e.g., almonds, walnuts), seeds (e.g., pumpkin seeds, sunflower seeds), unsweetened coconut flakes, granola (sugar-free or low-sugar)

Instructions:
1. In a blender, add the frozen berries, frozen banana, Greek yoghurt, almond milk, chia seeds or crushed flaxseed, cinnamon (optional), and spinach leaves.
2. Blend at high speeds until smooth and creamy. If the mixture is too thick, add a little more almond milk to get the right consistency.
3. After blending, pour the smoothie into a bowl.
4. Arrange the preferred toppings on top of the smoothie bowl.
5. Serve immediately and enjoy!

Veggie Breakfast Burrito

Ingredients:
- 4 large whole wheat or low-carb tortillas

- 8 large eggs
- 1 cup diced bell peppers (red, green, or yellow)
- 1 cup diced tomatoes
- 1 cup diced onions
- 1 cup diced mushrooms
- 1 cup spinach leaves
- 1/2 cup shredded low-fat cheddar cheese
- 1 tablespoon olive oil
- Salt and pepper to taste
- Optional: salsa, avocado slices, low-fat sour cream for serving

Instructions:

1. In a large skillet, heat olive oil over medium heat. Add the diced onions, bell peppers, and mushrooms. Sauté the vegetables for approximately 5-7 minutes, or until tender.
2. Add the diced tomatoes and spinach leaves to the skillet. Cook for 2-3 minutes, until the spinach has wilted and the tomatoes have softened. Season with salt and pepper to taste.
3. In a separate bowl, beat the eggs until thoroughly blended. Pour the beaten eggs into the skillet alongside the vegetables. Cook, stirring periodically, until the eggs are scrambled and cooked through, about 3-5 minutes.
4. To make the tortillas malleable, warm them in a dry skillet or in the microwave for a few seconds.
5. Divide the scrambled egg and vegetable mixture equally among the tortillas. Sprinkle shredded cheese on top of each serving.
6. To make burritos, fold the tortillas' sides over the filling and roll them tightly.

7. Warm the vegetable breakfast burritos and serve with salsa, avocado slices, or low-fat sour cream if desired.

Quinoa Breakfast Bowl

Ingredients :
- 1/2 cup quinoa, rinsed
- 1 cup water
- 1/2 teaspoon cinnamon
- 1/4 teaspoon ground nutmeg
- 1/4 teaspoon pure vanilla extract
- 1/2 cup unsweetened almond milk (or milk of choice)
- 1/2 cup fresh berries (such as strawberries, blueberries, or raspberries)
- 1 tablespoon chopped nuts (such as almonds, walnuts, or pecans)
- 1 tablespoon ground flaxseeds
- Optional: drizzle of honey or maple syrup (if desired)

Instructions:
1. In a small saucepan, combine the quinoa, water, cinnamon, nutmeg, and vanilla essence. Bring to a boil over medium high heat.
2. Reduce the heat to low, cover, and simmer for 15-20 minutes, or until the quinoa is cooked and the water has been absorbed.
3. Once cooked, fluff the quinoa with a fork and stir in the almond milk.
4. Divide the quinoa mixture across serving bowls.
5. Garnish each bowl with fresh berries, chopped almonds, and ground flaxseed.

6. Drizzle with honey or maple syrup for extra richness.
7. Serve warm and enjoy a nutritious start to your day!

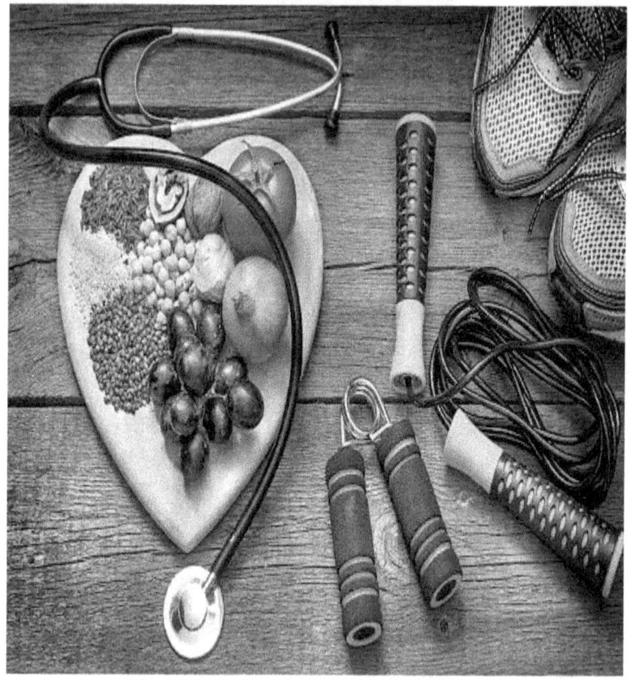

CHAPTER 2: LUNCH RECIPES

Grilled Chicken Salad

Ingredients :
- 2 boneless, skinless chicken breasts
- 4 cups mixed salad greens (such as spinach, arugula, and romaine)

- 1 cucumber, sliced
- 1 bell pepper, sliced
- 1 cup cherry tomatoes, halved
- 1/4 red onion, thinly sliced
- 1/4 cup sliced almonds
- 2 tablespoons olive oil
- 2 tablespoons balsamic vinegar
- Salt and pepper to taste

Instructions:

1. Preheat the grill to medium-high heat.
2. Season the chicken breasts with salt and pepper on both sides.
3. Place the chicken breasts on the hot grill and cook for 6-8 minutes per side, or until fully done and no longer pink in the centre. The cooking time may vary based on the thickness of the chicken breasts.
4. While the chicken is roasting, prepare the salad ingredients. In a large mixing bowl, add the salad greens, sliced cucumber, bell pepper, cherry tomatoes, red onion, and sliced almonds.
5. In a small mixing bowl, combine the olive oil and balsamic vinegar to prepare the dressing. Season with salt and pepper to taste.
6. When the chicken is fully cooked, remove it from the grill and let it rest for a few minutes. Next, slice the chicken breasts into thin strips.
7. Add the cut chicken to the salad bowl. Drizzle the dressing over the salad and gently toss to coat everything evenly.
8. Divide the salad among individual serving bowls or plates, and serve immediately.

Salmon with Roasted Vegetables

Ingredients:

- 4 salmon fillets (about 6 ounces each), skinless
- 2 tablespoons olive oil
- 2 cloves garlic, minced
- 1 teaspoon lemon zest
- 1 tablespoon lemon juice
- 1 teaspoon dried thyme
- Salt and pepper to taste
- 2 cups mixed vegetables (such as bell peppers, zucchini, cherry tomatoes, and red onions), chopped
- Cooking spray

Instructions:

1. Preheat the oven to 400 °F (200 °C).
2. In a small bowl, combine the olive oil, minced garlic, lemon zest, lemon juice, dried thyme, salt, and pepper.
3. Put the salmon fillets on a shallow plate and pour the olive oil mixture over them. Make sure the salmon is properly covered. Allow it to marinade for 15-20 minutes while you prepare the vegetables.
4. Line a baking sheet with parchment paper or aluminium foil, then gently cover with cooking spray.
5. Place the chopped vegetables on the prepared baking sheet. Drizzle with olive oil, then season with salt and pepper to taste. Toss the vegetables to properly distribute the oil and seasoning.
6. Arrange the marinated salmon fillets on a baking sheet alongside the vegetables.

7. Bake in the preheated oven for 15-20 minutes, or until the salmon is cooked through and easily flaked with a fork, and the veggies are soft and gently browned.
8. Remove from the oven and serve the salmon fillets alongside the roasted veggies.
9. Garnish with fresh herbs such as parsley or dill, and serve with a wedge of lemon on the side for added zest.
10. Enjoy your tasty and healthful salmon with roasted vegetables!

Quinoa and Black Bean Salad

Ingredients:
- 1 cup quinoa, rinsed
- 2 cups water or vegetable broth
- 1 can (15 ounces) black beans, drained and rinsed
- 1 cup cherry tomatoes, halved
- 1 bell pepper, diced (red, yellow, or green)
- 1/2 cup red onion, finely chopped
- 1/4 cup fresh cilantro, chopped
- 1 avocado, diced
- 1 lime, juiced
- 2 tablespoons olive oil
- Salt and pepper to taste

Instructions:
1. In a medium saucepan, heat the water or vegetable broth until it boils. Add the quinoa, decrease the heat to low, cover, and cook for 15 minutes, or until the liquid has been absorbed and the quinoa is soft. Remove from heat and allow to cool.

2. In a large mixing bowl, mix together the cooked quinoa, black beans, cherry tomatoes, bell pepper, red onion, and cilantro.
3. Make the dressing by whisking together lime juice, olive oil, salt, and pepper in a small bowl.
4. Toss the quinoa and black bean mixture slightly to coat with the dressing.
5. Gently fold in the cubed avocado.
6. Taste and adjust seasoning as needed.
7. Serve immediately or chill in the refrigerator for at least 30 minutes to enable the flavours to combine before serving.
8. Enjoy this delicious Quinoa and Black Bean Salad as a main course or as a side dish. It's high in protein, fibre, and minerals, making it a good choice for seniors with diabetes.

Turkey and Avocado Wrap

Ingredients:
- 4 whole wheat or whole grain tortillas (8-inch size)
- 8 slices of low-sodium deli turkey breast
- 1 ripe avocado, sliced
- 1 cup shredded lettuce
- 1/2 cup diced tomatoes
- 1/4 cup thinly sliced red onion
- 1/4 cup sliced cucumber
- 1/4 cup plain Greek yogurt (low-fat or fat-free)
- 1 tablespoon Dijon mustard
- 1 tablespoon lemon juice
- Salt and pepper to taste

Instructions:

1. Arrange the tortillas on a clean surface.
2. In a small bowl, combine the Greek yoghurt and Dijon mustard. Spread the mixture evenly on each tortilla.
3. Place two slices of turkey breast on each tortilla, leaving room around the borders.
4. Spread the avocado slices, spinach leaves, cucumber slices, chopped tomatoes, and sliced red onion evenly across the turkey.
5. Season with salt and pepper to taste.
6. Starting at one end, tightly roll each tortilla into a wrap.
7. Cut each wrap in half diagonally to serve, or leave whole for a bigger serving.
8. Serve right away, or wrap each individual wrap in parchment paper or aluminium foil for easy transportation or storage.

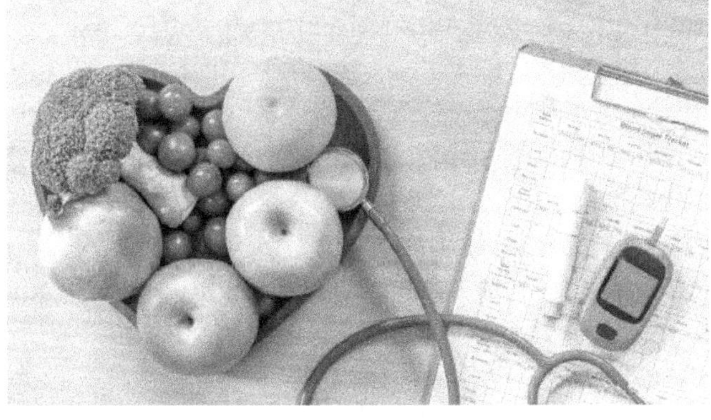

Mushroom and Spinach Frittata

Ingredients:
- 8 large eggs
- 1 cup sliced mushrooms
- 2 cups fresh spinach leaves, roughly chopped

- 1 small onion, diced
- 2 cloves garlic, minced
- 1 tablespoon olive oil
- Salt and pepper to taste
- 1/4 cup shredded low-fat cheese (optional)

Instructions:

1. Preheat the oven grill.
2. In a large oven-safe skillet, heat the olive oil over medium heat. Combine the diced onion and minced garlic. Sauté until the onion is transparent and the garlic is aromatic, about 2-3 minutes.
3. Add the sliced mushrooms to the skillet. Cook until the mushrooms are soft and any liquid has evaporated, which should take around 5-7 minutes.
4. Add the chopped spinach to the skillet. Cook for approximately 2-3 minutes, or until the spinach has wilted. Season with salt and pepper to taste.
5. In a mixing bowl, whisk the eggs until thoroughly combined. Pour the beaten eggs onto the mushroom and spinach mixture in the skillet. Gently stir to incorporate, making sure the vegetables are well dispersed among the eggs.
6. Cook the frittata over medium heat, without stirring, until the edges start to set, about 5 minutes.
7. If using cheese, sprinkle it evenly over the frittata.
8. Place the skillet under the preheated oven grill. Broil the frittata for approximately 3-5 minutes, or until the top is set and golden brown. Keep a tight eye on it to avoid scorching.

9. Once finished, remove the skillet from the oven. Let the frittata cool slightly before slicing it into wedges.

10. Serve the Mushroom and Spinach Frittata warm or room temperature. Enjoy this delicious and nutritious dinner that is ideal for a diabetic diet.

Turkey and Veggie Skewers

Ingredients:
- 1 pound turkey breast, cut into 1-inch cubes
- 2 bell peppers (red, green, or yellow), cut into chunks
- 1 large red onion, cut into chunks
- 8-10 cherry tomatoes
- 8-10 button mushrooms, cleaned
- 2 tablespoons olive oil
- 2 cloves garlic, minced
- 1 teaspoon dried oregano
- 1 teaspoon dried thyme
- Salt and pepper to taste
- Wooden or metal skewers

Instructions:
1. Soak wooden skewers in water for at least 30 minutes to avoid scorching during grilling.
2. In a mixing dish, combine olive oil, minced garlic, dried oregano, dried thyme, salt, and pepper. Mix thoroughly to make a marinade.
3. Place the turkey breast cubes in the marinade, making sure they are thoroughly coated. Allow it to marinade for at least 30 minutes, preferably overnight in the refrigerator.
4. Preheat the grill to medium-high heat.

5. While the grill is cooking, thread the marinated turkey cubes, bell peppers, onions, cherry tomatoes, and mushrooms onto the skewers in alternate order.
6. After assembling the skewers, carefully coat them with any residual marinade.
7. Place the skewers on the hot grill and cook for approximately 10-15 minutes, Turn the turkey occasionally until it's fully cooked and the vegetables are soft and slightly browned.
8. Remove the skewers from the grill and allow them rest for a few minutes before serving.
9. Serve the turkey and vegetable skewers hot with brown rice or quinoa for a well-balanced meal that is ideal for a diabetic diet.

Cauliflower Crust Pizza

Ingredients:
- 1 medium head of cauliflower
- 1/2 cup shredded mozzarella cheese
- 1/4 cup grated Parmesan cheese
- 1/2 teaspoon dried oregano
- 1/2 teaspoon garlic powder
- 1/4 teaspoon salt
- 1/4 teaspoon black pepper
- 1 egg, beaten
- 1/4 cup marinara sauce (look for low-sugar options)
- 1/2 cup shredded part-skim mozzarella cheese
- Desired pizza toppings (e.g., vegetables, lean meats)

Instructions:

1. Preheat the oven to 400 °F (200 °C). Line a baking sheet with parchment paper.
2. Wash the cauliflower and remove its core. Cut the cauliflower into florets and pulse them in a food processor until they are fine crumbs. Alternatively, grate the cauliflower with a box grater.
3. Place the cauliflower crumbs in a microwave-safe basin and heat on high for 5-6 minutes, or until soft. Let it cool for a few minutes.
4. Once cooled, place the cauliflower crumbs on a clean kitchen towel or cheesecloth. Squeeze as much moisture as possible. This step is essential for achieving a crispy crust.
5. In a mixing bowl, combine the squeezed cauliflower, shredded mozzarella, Parmesan, dried oregano, garlic powder, salt, black pepper, and beaten egg. Mix until thoroughly mixed.
6. Transfer the cauliflower mixture on the prepared baking sheet. Using your hands, press and form the dough into a thin, spherical crust approximately 1/4 inch thick. Make the edges slightly thicker to resemble the crust.
7. Bake the cauliflower crust in a preheated oven for 20-25 minutes, until golden brown and firm to the touch.
8. When the crust is finished, take it from the oven and spread the marinara sauce evenly over the top, leaving a little border around the borders.
9. Sprinkle shredded mozzarella cheese over the sauce and top with your preferred pizza toppings.

10. Return the pizza to the oven and cook for another 10-12 minutes, or until the cheese is melted and bubbling.
11. Remove the pizza from the oven and allow to cool for a few minutes before slicing and serving.

Tuna Salad Lettuce Wraps

Ingredients:
- 2 cans (5 ounces each) of water-packed tuna, drained
- 1/4 cup light mayonnaise
- 1 tablespoon Dijon mustard
- 2 celery stalks, finely chopped
- 1/4 cup red onion, finely chopped
- 1/4 cup dill pickles, finely chopped
- 1 tablespoon fresh lemon juice
- Salt and pepper to taste
- 8 large lettuce leaves (such as romaine or iceberg)
- Optional: cherry tomatoes for garnish

Instructions:
1. In a medium mixing bowl, combine the drained tuna, light mayonnaise, Dijon mustard, chopped celery, red onion, dill pickles, and lemon juice. Mix thoroughly until all components are uniformly distributed.
2. Season the tuna salad with salt and pepper to taste. If desired, adjust the lemon juice and mustard.
3. Wash and dry the lettuce leaves well. To eliminate any excess moisture, pat them dry with paper towels.
4. Arrange the lettuce leaves on a clean, flat surface.

5. Distribute the tuna salad mixture evenly among the lettuce leaves.
6. Gently roll up each lettuce leaf, securing the tuna salad filling inside.
7. If preferred, top each lettuce wrap with a cherry tomato for extra flavour and appeal.
8. Serve immediately and enjoy your tasty and healthful Tuna Salad Lettuce Wraps!

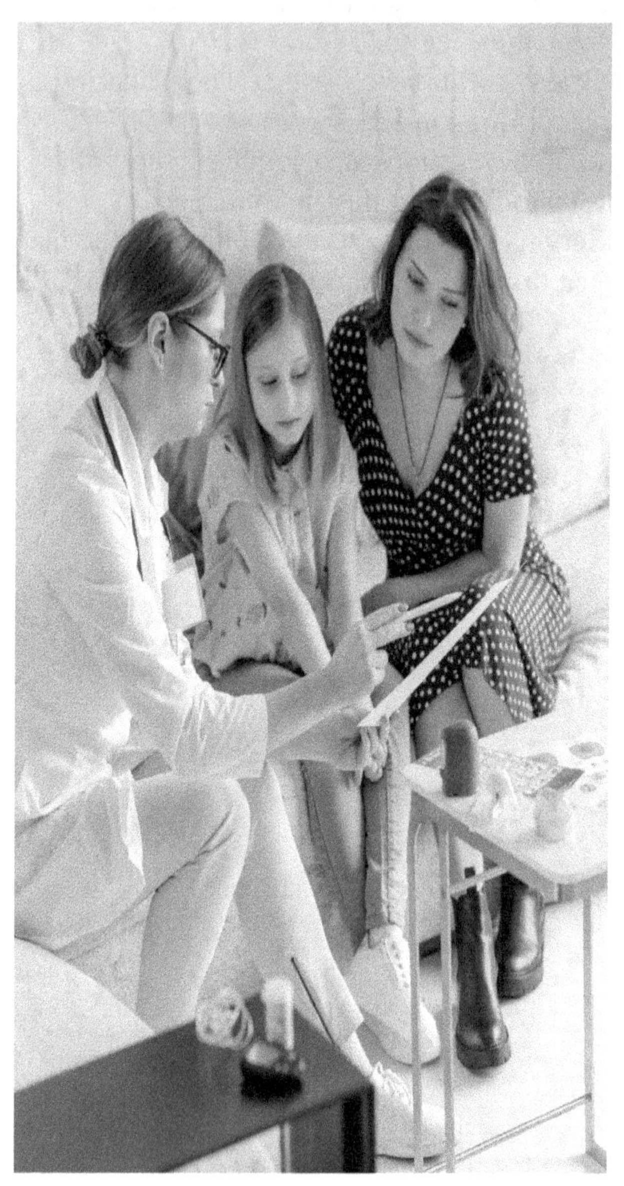

CHAPTER 3: DINNER RECIPES

Grilled Salmon with Asparagus

Ingredients:
- 4 salmon fillets, skin-on, about 6 ounces each
- 1 bunch of asparagus, trimmed
- 2 tablespoons olive oil
- 2 cloves garlic, minced
- 1 teaspoon lemon zest
- 2 tablespoons fresh lemon juice
- Salt and pepper to taste
- Fresh chopped parsley for garnish

Instructions:
1. Preheat the grill to medium-high heat. Make sure the grill grates are clean and gently greased to avoid sticking.
2. In a small bowl, combine olive oil, minced garlic, lemon zest, and lemon juice to make a marinade.
3. Place the salmon fillets and the trimmed asparagus spears in separate shallow bowls. Pour half of the marinade over the salmon fillets, and the other half over the asparagus. Gently toss to provide a uniform coating. Allow them to marinade for approximately 15-20 minutes at room temperature.
4. Once marinated, take the salmon fillets from the marinade and shake off the excess. Season both sides of the salmon fillets with salt and pepper to taste.
5. Place the salmon fillets skin side down on the preheated grill. Grill for about 4-5 minutes per

side, or until the salmon is fully cooked and readily flaked with a fork.

6. While the salmon cooks, set the marinated asparagus spears directly on the grill. Grill for 3-4 minutes, flipping regularly, until tender and gently browned.

7. When the salmon and asparagus are done, remove them from the grill and place on a serving plate.

8. If preferred, garnish the grilled salmon and asparagus with freshly chopped parsley and more lemon wedges.

9. For a tasty and nutritious lunch, pair the grilled salmon with asparagus and your favourite side dish, such as brown rice or quinoa .

Turkey and Vegetable Stir-Fry

Ingredients:
- 1 lb lean turkey breast, thinly sliced
- 2 tablespoons olive oil
- 2 cloves garlic, minced
- 1 onion, sliced
- 2 cups broccoli florets
- 1 red bell pepper, sliced
- 1 yellow bell pepper, sliced
- 1 cup snow peas, trimmed
- 2 carrots, julienned
- 1/4 cup low-sodium soy sauce
- 2 tablespoons rice vinegar
- 1 tablespoon honey or sugar substitute (optional)
- 1 teaspoon sesame oil
- 1 teaspoon ginger, grated
- Salt and pepper to taste
- Cooked brown rice or quinoa, for serving (optional)

Instructions:

1. In a small mixing bowl, combine the soy sauce, rice vinegar, honey (or sugar substitute), sesame oil, and shredded ginger. Set aside.
2. Heat 1 tablespoon olive oil in a large skillet or wok over medium-high heat. Stir-fry the sliced turkey breast for 5-6 minutes, or until thoroughly done. Remove the turkey from the skillet and set it aside.
3. In the same skillet, heat the remaining tablespoon olive oil. Stir add the minced garlic and chopped onion, cooking for 2-3 minutes until aromatic and softened.
4. Add the broccoli florets, sliced bell peppers, snow peas, and julienned carrots to the skillet. Stir-fry for another 4-5 minutes, until the vegetables are soft and crunchy.
5. Return the cooked turkey to the skillet alongside the veggies. Pour the prepared sauce over the turkey and vegetables, stirring to cover. Cook for another 2-3 minutes, until everything has heated through and the sauce has thickened somewhat.
6. Season with salt and pepper to taste.
7. If desired, serve the turkey and veggie stir-fry hot with cooked brown rice or quinoa.

Quinoa Stuffed Bell Peppers

Ingredients:

- 4 large bell peppers (any color)
- 1 cup quinoa, rinsed
- 2 cups vegetable broth
- 1 small onion, finely chopped

- 2 cloves garlic, minced
- 1 can (15 ounces) diced tomatoes, drained
- 1 cup cooked black beans, drained and rinsed
- 1 cup cooked corn kernels
- 1 teaspoon ground cumin
- 1 teaspoon smoked paprika
- Salt and pepper to taste
- 1/2 cup shredded cheddar cheese (optional)
- Fresh cilantro, chopped, for garnish

Instructions:

1. Preheat the oven to 375°F (190° C).
2. Cut the bell pepper tops off and remove the seeds and membranes. Set aside.
3. In a medium saucepan, mix the quinoa with the vegetable broth. Bring to a boil, then reduce to a low heat, cover, and simmer for 15 minutes, or until the quinoa is cooked and the liquid has been absorbed.
4. In a big skillet, heat a little olive oil over medium heat. Sauté the chopped onion and garlic until softened, about 3-4 minutes.
5. Add the chopped tomatoes, black beans, corn kernels, cumin, smoked paprika, salt and pepper to the pan. Stir to blend and simmer for an additional 5 minutes.
6. When the quinoa is done, add it to the skillet with the veggie mixture. Stir thoroughly to mix.
7. Fill each bell pepper with the quinoa and veggie mixture, gently pressing down to compact it in.
8. Transfer the stuffed peppers to a baking dish. If using cheese, add it on top of the stuffed peppers.
9. Cover the baking dish with foil and bake for 25-30 minutes, until the peppers are cooked.

10. Remove the foil and continue baking for 5-10 minutes, or until the cheese is melted and bubbling (if using).
11. Remove from the oven and allow it cool for a few minutes before serving.
12. Garnish with chopped fresh cilantro before serving.

Chicken and Vegetable Skewers :

Ingredients:
- 1 lb boneless, skinless chicken breasts, cut into chunks
- 1 red bell pepper, cut into chunks
- 1 green bell pepper, cut into chunks
- 1 yellow onion, cut into chunks
- 8 cherry tomatoes
- 8 button mushrooms, cleaned
- 2 tablespoons olive oil
- 2 cloves garlic, minced
- 1 teaspoon dried oregano
- 1 teaspoon dried thyme
- Salt and pepper to taste
- Wooden skewers, soaked in water for 30 minutes

Instructions:
1. Preheat your grill to medium-high, or your oven to 400°F (200°C) if you want to bake.
2. In a small bowl, combine olive oil, minced garlic, dried oregano, dried thyme, salt, and pepper to make a marinade.
3. Put the chicken chunks in a big basin and pour the marinade over them. To get an equal coating,

toss the chicken thoroughly. Allow to marinate for at least 20 minutes in the refrigerator.
4. While the chicken is marinating, chop the vegetables into bits.
5. Thread the marinated chicken, bell peppers, onion, cherry tomatoes, and mushrooms on the soaked wooden skewers, alternating them.
6. If grilling, lightly oil the grill grate before grilling the skewers for 10-12 minutes, rotating regularly, until the chicken is fully cooked and the vegetables are soft.
7. If baking, set the skewers on a baking sheet coated with parchment paper and bake for 20-25 minutes, or until the chicken is fully cooked and the vegetables are soft.
8. Serve the chicken and veggie skewers hot, either alone or with a side of brown rice or quinoa for a complete dinner .

Baked Cod with Roasted Vegetables

Ingredients:
- 4 cod fillets (6 ounces each)
- 2 tablespoons olive oil
- 2 cloves garlic, minced
- 1 teaspoon dried thyme
- 1 teaspoon dried oregano
- Salt and pepper to taste
- 2 cups mixed vegetables (such as bell peppers, zucchini, and cherry tomatoes), chopped
- 1 lemon, sliced
- Fresh parsley, chopped (for garnish)

Instructions

1. Preheat the oven to 400 °F (200 °C). Line a baking sheet with parchment paper or lightly coat it with olive oil.
2. In a small bowl, combine the olive oil, minced garlic, dried thyme, dried oregano, salt, and pepper.
3. Place the fish fillets on the prepared baking sheet. Brush each fillet with the olive oil mixture, ensuring that both sides are coated.
4. Toss the mixed veggies in a big bowl with the remaining olive oil mixture until well coated.
5. Place the vegetables around the fish fillets on the baking sheet. Place lemon wedges on top of each cod fillet.
6. Bake in the preheated oven for 15-20 minutes, or until the cod is cooked through and easily flaked with a fork, and the veggies are soft and gently browned.
7. Once finished, remove from the oven and allow it cool for a few minutes. Before serving, garnish with finely chopped fresh parsley.
8. Serve the baked cod with roasted veggies hot for a tasty and healthful supper !

Zucchini Noodles with Turkey Meatballs

Ingredients:
- 4 medium zucchinis, spiralized into noodles
- 1 pound lean ground turkey
- 1/4 cup whole wheat breadcrumbs
- 1/4 cup grated Parmesan cheese
- 1 egg

- 2 cloves garlic, minced
- 1 teaspoon dried oregano
- 1/2 teaspoon dried basil
- 1/2 teaspoon salt
- 1/4 teaspoon black pepper
- 2 tablespoons olive oil
- 1 can (14 ounces) crushed tomatoes
- 1 teaspoon dried parsley
- Grated Parmesan cheese, for serving (optional)
- Fresh basil leaves, for garnish (optional)

Instructions:

1. In a large mixing bowl, combine the ground turkey, breadcrumbs, grated Parmesan cheese, egg, chopped garlic, dried oregano and basil, salt, and black pepper. Mix until thoroughly mixed.
2. Shape the turkey mixture into meatballs approximately an inch in diameter.
3. In a large skillet, warm 1 tablespoon olive oil over medium heat. Cook the turkey meatballs in the skillet, turning regularly, until browned on both sides and cooked through, about 10 to 12 minutes. Remove the meatballs from the skillet and set them aside.
4. In the same skillet, heat the remaining tablespoon olive oil. Add the spiralized zucchini noodles to the skillet and cook for 2-3 minutes, or until just soft but still crunchy.
5. Pour the smashed tomatoes onto the zucchini noodles in the skillet. Stir in the dry parsley until thoroughly combined. Let the sauce simmer for 2-3 minutes.
6. Return the cooked turkey meatballs to the skillet alongside the zucchini noodles and tomato sauce.

Gently combine everything until the meatballs are heated through.

7. Serve the zucchini noodles and turkey meatballs hot, topped with grated Parmesan cheese and fresh basil leaves, if desired .

Salad Nicoise

Ingredients:
- 2 cups mixed salad greens (such as lettuce, spinach, and arugula)
- 1 cup cherry tomatoes, halved
- 1/2 cup cooked green beans, trimmed
- 1/2 cup canned tuna in water, drained
- 2 hard-boiled eggs, peeled and quartered
- 1/4 cup sliced black olives (preferably low-sodium)
- 2 tablespoons chopped fresh parsley
- 1 tablespoon capers, rinsed and drained
- 1 tablespoon extra-virgin olive oil
- 1 tablespoon red wine vinegar
- Salt and pepper to taste

Instructions:
1. Begin by placing the mixed salad greens on a big serving platter or individual plates.
2. Spread the halved cherry tomatoes and cooked green beans over the salad greens.
3. Add the drained canned tuna to the salad and distribute it evenly.
4. Arrange the quartered hard-boiled eggs around the salad.
5. Sprinkle the sliced black olives and capers on top of the salad.

6. Make the dressing by whisking together extra-virgin olive oil and red wine vinegar in a small bowl. Season with salt and pepper to taste.
7. Drizzle the dressing on the Salad Niçoise right before serving.
8. Garnish with chopped fresh parsley for extra flavour and presentation.
9. Serve immediately and enjoy this healthful and delicious Salad Niçoise designed just for elderly diabetics.

Vegetable and Tofu Stir-Fry

Ingredients:
- 1 block firm tofu, drained and cubed
- 2 tablespoons low-sodium soy sauce
- 2 tablespoons olive oil
- 2 cloves garlic, minced
- 1 tablespoon fresh ginger, minced
- 1 onion, thinly sliced
- 2 carrots, julienned
- 1 red bell pepper, thinly sliced
- 1 cup broccoli florets
- 1 cup snap peas, trimmed
- 1 cup mushrooms, sliced
- 2 cups cooked brown rice or quinoa
- Salt and pepper to taste
- Optional garnishes: sesame seeds, green onions

Instructions:
1. To drain extra moisture from the tofu, wrap it in paper towels and set it on top of something heavy. Allow it to settle for approximately 15-20 minutes.

2. In a small bowl, combine the soy sauce, minced garlic, and ginger. Set aside.
3. Heat 1 tablespoon olive oil in a large skillet or wok over medium-high heat. Cook the tofu cubes till golden brown on all sides, which should take about 5-7 minutes. Remove the tofu from the skillet and set it aside.
4. In the same skillet, heat the remaining tablespoon olive oil. Cook the sliced onion until transparent, about 2-3 minutes.
5. Add the carrots, bell pepper, broccoli, snap peas, and mushrooms to the pan. Stir-fry for 5-7 minutes, or until the vegetables are soft and crispy.
6. Return the tofu to the skillet, then pour the soy sauce mixture over the vegetables. Stir thoroughly to incorporate and coat everything evenly. Cook for a another 2–3 minutes.
7. Season with salt and pepper to taste.
8. Serve the vegetable and tofu stir-fry with cooked brown rice or quinoa.
9. If desired, garnish with sesame seeds and thinly sliced green onions.
10. Enjoy your nutritious and delicious vegetable and tofu stir-fry, specifically designed to help seniors manage their diabetes !

Spaghetti Squash with Turkey Bolognese

Ingredients:
- 1 medium spaghetti squash
- 1 lb lean ground turkey
- 1 tablespoon olive oil

- 1 small onion, finely chopped
- 2 cloves garlic, minced
- 1 carrot, finely chopped
- 1 celery stalk, finely chopped
- 1 can (14 oz) diced tomatoes
- 1 can (6 oz) tomato paste
- 1 teaspoon dried oregano
- 1 teaspoon dried basil
- Salt and pepper to taste
- Grated Parmesan cheese for garnish (optional)
- Fresh basil leaves for garnish (optional)

Instructions:

1. Preheat the oven to 400 °F (200 °C).
2. Cut the spaghetti squash in half lengthwise, then scoop out the seeds with a spoon. Place the squash halves, cut side down, on a baking sheet covered with parchment paper. Bake in the preheated oven for 40-50 minutes, or until the squash is soft and readily penetrated by a fork.
3. While the squash is baking, warm the olive oil in a large skillet over medium heat. Combine the diced onion, garlic, carrot, and celery. Cook, stirring occasionally, until the veggies have softened, about 5-7 minutes.
4. Place the lean ground turkey in the skillet with the veggies. Cook for 8-10 minutes, breaking the turkey up with a spoon while it cooks.
5. Combine the chopped tomatoes, tomato paste, dry oregano, and dried basil. Season with salt and pepper to taste. Reduce the heat to low and let the sauce simmer for 15-20 minutes, letting the flavours to combine.

6. Once the spaghetti squash is cooked, take it from the oven and allow it to cool slightly. Use a fork to scrape the squash flesh into strands that resemble spaghetti noodles.
7. Divide the spaghetti squash noodles among serving plates, then top with the turkey bolognese.
8. If preferred, garnish with grated Parmesan cheese and fresh basil leaves just before serving .

CHAPTER 4: DESSERTS AND TREATS

Sugar-Free Berry Parfait

Ingredients:
- 1 cup of mixed berries (such as strawberries, blueberries, raspberries)
- 1 cup of plain Greek yogurt (unsweetened)
- 1/2 teaspoon of vanilla extract
- 1/4 cup of chopped nuts (such as almonds, walnuts) for garnish (optional)
- Fresh mint leaves for garnish (optional)

Instructions:
1. **Prepare the Berries:**
    - Wash the berries thoroughly in cold water before patting them dry with a paper towel.
    - If using strawberries, remove the stems and cut into small pieces. Leave the smaller berries whole.
2. **Prepare the Yogurt:**

- In a mixing dish, add plain Greek yoghurt and vanilla extract. Mix thoroughly until the vanilla is uniformly dispersed throughout the yoghurt.

3. **Assemble the Parfaits:**
   - Grab two serving glasses or bowls.
   - Begin layering the parfait by spooning a dollop of vanilla yoghurt into the bottom of each glass, being sure to cover the base equally .

4. **Add the Berries:**
   - Place a layer of mixed berries on top of the yoghurt. Distribute the berries equally over the yoghurt layer. .

5. **Repeat Layers:**
   - Continue layering with another spoonful of vanilla yoghurt, then another layer of berries, until all of the ingredients have been utilised. Ensure that the top layer is yoghurt.

6. **Garnish:**
   - If preferred, put chopped nuts on top of each parfait for texture and flavour.
   - To add a beautiful touch, garnish with fresh mint leaves.

7. **Chill and Serve:**
   - Refrigerate the constructed parfaits for at least 30 minutes before serving. Chilling helps the flavours blend together.
   - Serve the sugar-free berry parfaits cooled for a delightful and nutritious dessert or snack .

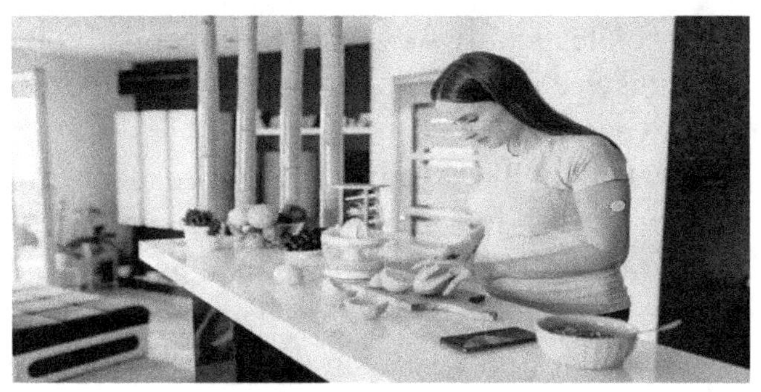

Dark Chocolate-Dipped Strawberries

Ingredients:
- 1 pint fresh strawberries, rinsed and dried thoroughly
- 4 ounces dark chocolate (at least 70% cocoa), chopped
- 1 teaspoon coconut oil
- Optional toppings: chopped nuts (such as almonds or walnuts), unsweetened coconut flakes

Instructions:
1. Line a baking sheet with parchment paper or a silicone baking mat.
2. In a microwave-safe bowl, mix together the chopped dark chocolate and coconut oil. Microwave the chocolate in 30-second intervals, stirring between each, until it is melted and smooth. Take care not to overheat the chocolate.
3. Dip each strawberry by the stem into the melted chocolate, swirling to cover about two-thirds of the strawberry. Allow the extra chocolate to trickle off.
4. Place the chocolate-dipped strawberries on the prepared baking sheet. If desired, while the

chocolate is still wet, sprinkle chopped almonds or unsweetened coconut flakes over the dipped strawberries.
5. Once all of the strawberries have been dipped, place the baking sheet in the refrigerator for 15-20 minutes, or until the chocolate has hardened.
6. Once the chocolate has hardened, place the strawberries on a serving dish or container. If not serving immediately, refrigerate the chocolate-dipped strawberries until ready to serve.
7. Enjoy these delectable delicacies in moderation as part of a healthy diabetes diet. Remember to account for the carbohydrate content of the strawberries and alter insulin or medication doses as needed.

Baked Apples with Cinnamon

Ingredients:
- 4 medium-sized apples (choose varieties like Gala, Fuji, or Granny Smith)
- 2 tablespoons unsalted butter, melted
- 2 teaspoons ground cinnamon
- 2 tablespoons sugar substitute (such as erythritol or stevia)
- 1/4 cup chopped walnuts (optional)
- 1/4 cup raisins (optional)
- 1/4 cup water

Instructions:
1. Preheat the oven to 350°F (175° C). Coat a baking dish lightly with butter or nonstick cooking spray.

2. Wash the apples thoroughly with running water. Dry them with a clean kitchen towel.
3. Core each apple gently, removing the seeds and making a well in the centre for the filling. You can use an apple corer or a sharp knife to accomplish this.
4. In a small bowl, blend the melted butter, ground cinnamon, and sugar substitute until well incorporated. Sweetness can be adjusted to suit individual taste preferences and dietary requirements.
5. If using, combine the chopped walnuts and raisins with the cinnamon mixture.
6. Put the cored apples in a greased baking tray. Spoon the cinnamon mixture equally into the centre of each apple, filling it completely.
7. Pour the water into the bottom of the baking dish. The water will help to generate steam and keep the apples from drying out during baking.
8. Cover the baking dish with aluminium foil and place in the preheated oven.
9. Bake the apples for 30 to 40 minutes, or until soft. To test for doneness, poke a fork into the apples; they should easily penetrate.
10. Once baked, remove the foil from the baking dish and allow the apples to cool before serving.
11. To add flavour, top the baked apples with a dollop of Greek yoghurt or a sprinkle of cinnamon.
12. Enjoy these delicious and diabetes-friendly baked apples with cinnamon as a healthful dessert or snack!

Greek Yogurt Popsicles

Ingredients:
- 2 cups plain Greek yogurt (low-fat or non-fat)
- 1 cup mixed berries (such as blueberries, raspberries, and strawberries), fresh or frozen
- 2 tablespoons honey or agave syrup (optional, depending on sweetness preference)
- 1 teaspoon vanilla extract (optional)
- Popsicle molds
- Popsicle sticks

Instructions:
1. **Prepare the Berries:**
   - If using fresh berries, thoroughly rinse them under cold water before patting them dry with a paper towel.
   - If using frozen berries, let them thaw at room temperature for a few minutes.
2. **Blend the Berries:**
   - In a blender or food processor, combine the berries. Pulse a few times to roughly chop and mash the berries, but keep them chunky. You can also purée them for a smoother texture.
3. **Sweeten the Yogurt:**
   - In a mixing bowl, whisk together the Greek yoghurt, honey or agave syrup (if using), and vanilla extract. Mix vigorously until the sugar is completely mixed into the yoghurt.
4. **Layering:**
   - Layer the Greek yoghurt mixture and mashed berries in popsicle moulds

alternately. Begin with a teaspoon of yoghurt, then add a spoonful of berries, and repeat until the moulds are full.

5. **Insert Popsicle Sticks:**
   - Once the moulds are full, lightly tap them on the counter to remove any air bubbles and ensure that the mixture settles evenly. Place the popsicle sticks in the centre of each mould.

6. **Freezing:**
   - Place the popsicle moulds in the freezer for at least 4-6 hours, or until fully frozen.

7. **Unmolding:**
   - When you're ready to serve, take the popsicle moulds from the freezer. To remove the popsicles from the moulds, run warm water over the outside for a few seconds to loosen them. Gently tug on the sticks to release the popsicles.

8. **Serve and Enjoy:**
   - Serve the Greek yoghurt popsicles right away and enjoy the delicious delight. Keep any leftover popsicles in an airtight jar in the freezer for up to two weeks.

Almond Flour Cookies

Ingredients:
- 2 cups almond flour
- 1/4 cup coconut oil, melted
- 1/4 cup natural sweetener (such as erythritol or stevia)

- 1 teaspoon vanilla extract
- 1/4 teaspoon salt
- 1/4 teaspoon baking soda
- 1/3 cup sugar-free dark chocolate chips (optional)
- Chopped nuts (optional, for added texture)

Instructions:

1. Preheat the oven to 350°F (175° C). Line a baking sheet with parchment paper or lightly grease it with coconut oil to keep it from sticking.
2. In a large mixing bowl, add almond flour, melted coconut oil, natural sweetener, vanilla extract, salt, and baking soda. Stir until thoroughly incorporated and dough forms.
3. If desired, add sugar-free dark chocolate chips or chopped almonds to the dough for extra flavour and texture.
4. Use a spoon or cookie scoop to portion out the dough and roll it into balls. Place the balls on the prepared baking sheet, leaving some space between each cookie because they will spread somewhat during baking.
5. Use a fork to carefully flatten each cookie ball, leaving a crisscross design on top.
6. Bake the cookies in the preheated oven for 10-12 minutes, or until golden brown around the edges.
7. Remove the cookies from the oven and cool for a few minutes on the baking sheet before transferring to a wire rack to finish cooling.
8. Once chilled, keep the almond flour cookies in an airtight container at room temperature for up to a week. Enjoy them as a tasty, diabetic-friendly treat!

Chia Seed Pudding

Ingredients:
- 1/2 cup chia seeds
- 2 cups unsweetened almond milk (or any unsweetened milk of choice)
- 1 teaspoon vanilla extract
- 1-2 tablespoons sweetener (stevia, erythritol, or any preferred sugar substitute)
- Fresh berries or nuts for topping (optional)

Instructions:
1. **Mix Ingredients:** In a mixing bowl, blend chia seeds, unsweetened almond milk, vanilla extract, and sweetener. Stir until everything is well combined. Allow the mixture to sit for 5 minutes before stirring again to avoid clumping.
2. **Refrigerate overnight:** by covering the mixing basin with plastic wrap or transferring the mixture to individual serving cups. Refrigerate the mixture for at least 4 hours, preferably overnight, to allow the chia seeds to absorb the liquid and thicken.
3. **Stir before serving:** mix the pudding thoroughly to properly distribute the chia seeds. If the custard is too thick, add a splash of almond milk to achieve the appropriate consistency.
4. **Add Toppings:** Serve the chia seed pudding in individual dishes or cups. If preferred, garnish with fresh berries, nuts, or a dusting of cinnamon. These toppings enhance the dessert's flavour and texture while keeping it diabetes-friendly.
5. **Enjoy:** Serve the chia seed pudding cooled for a wonderful, diabetes-friendly dessert or snack!

Frozen Banana Bites

Ingredients:
- 2 large ripe bananas
- 1/4 cup dark chocolate chips (at least 70% cocoa)
- 1/4 cup unsweetened shredded coconut
- 1/4 cup finely chopped nuts (such as almonds, walnuts, or peanuts)
- Parchment paper

Instructions:
1. **Prepare the Bananas:**
   - Cut the bananas into 1-inch slices and lay them on a parchment-lined baking sheet.
   - To avoid sticking together, make sure the banana slices do not contact.
2. **Spread Nut Butter:**
   - With a small spoon or knife, apply a thin coating of almond or peanut butter on top of each banana slice.
3. **Freeze:**
   - Place the baking sheet containing the banana slices in the freezer for at least one hour, or until hard.
4. **Prepare Chocolate Coating:**
   - In a microwave-safe bowl, mix together the dark chocolate chips and coconut oil.
   - Microwave for 30-second intervals, stirring in between, until the chocolate is melted and smooth.
5. **Coat the Bananas:**
   - Remove the frozen banana slices from the freezer.

- Using a fork or toothpick, evenly coat each banana slice in the melted chocolate.
- Allow any extra chocolate to drip off before returning the coated banana bite to the parchment-lined baking sheet.

6. **Optional Toppings:**
   - Before the chocolate hardens, sprinkle chopped almonds, shredded coconut, or chia seeds over the covered banana bites.

7. **Final Freeze:**
   - Once all of the banana pieces are coated and topped, place the baking sheet in the freezer.
   - Allow the banana bits to freeze for at least one additional hour, or until the chocolate coating is completely set.

8. **Serve:**
   - Once the banana bites are completely frozen, place them in an airtight container or zip-top bag to keep in the freezer.
   - These frozen banana bites are a tasty and refreshing treat that can be eaten straight from the freezer.

Coconut Flour Muffins

Ingredients:
- 1/2 cup coconut flour
- 1/4 cup unsweetened shredded coconut
- 1/2 teaspoon baking powder
- 1/4 teaspoon salt
- 4 large eggs
- 1/4 cup coconut oil, melted

- 1/4 cup unsweetened almond milk (or any milk alternative)
- 1/4 cup natural sweetener (such as erythritol or stevia), adjust to taste
- 1 teaspoon vanilla extract
- Optional: 1/4 cup chopped nuts (such as pecans or walnuts) for added texture.

Instructions:

1. Preheat the oven to 350°F (175° C). Grease a muffin tray or use paper liners.
2. In a mixing basin, whisk together the coconut flour, shredded coconut, baking powder, and salt. Mix thoroughly to ensure there are no lumps.
3. In a separate bowl, mix the eggs, melted coconut oil, almond milk, natural sweetener, and vanilla essence until thoroughly blended.
4. Gradually combine the wet and dry ingredients, stirring until the batter is smooth and well combined. If desired, mix in the chopped nuts.
5. Spoon the batter evenly into the prepared muffin cups, filling them about 3/4 full.
6. Bake the muffins in the preheated oven for 20-25 minutes, or until golden brown and a toothpick inserted into the centre comes clean.
7. Let the muffins cool in the tin for a few minutes before transferring them to a wire rack to finish cooling.
8. Serve and enjoy these delectable coconut flour muffins as a nutritious snack or breakfast choice for seniors on a diabetes-friendly diet

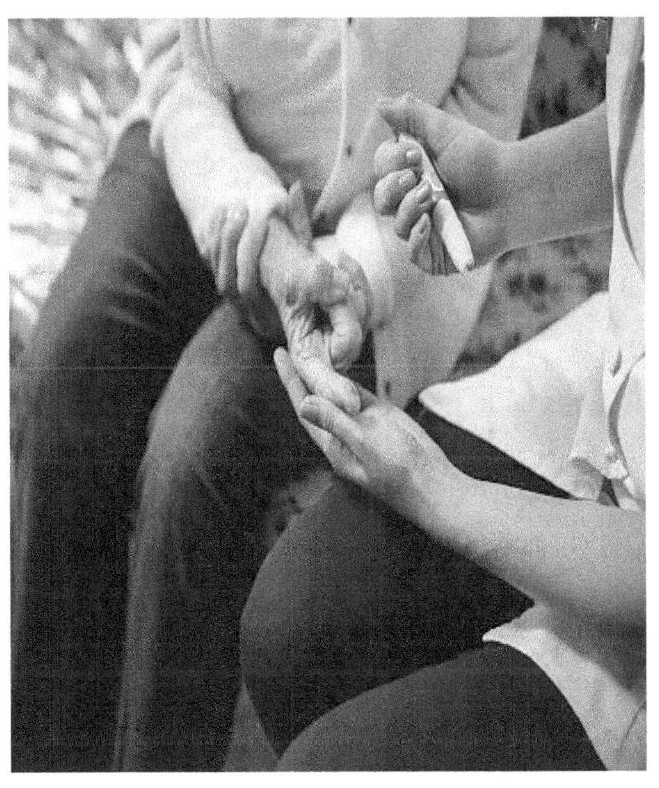

CHAPTER 5: SNACKS AND APPETIZERS

Cucumber Slices with Cottage Cheese

Ingredients:
- 2 medium cucumbers, washed and thinly sliced
- 1 cup low-fat cottage cheese
- 1 tablespoon fresh dill, finely chopped
- 1 tablespoon fresh chives, finely chopped

- 1 tablespoon lemon juice
- Salt and pepper to taste

Instructions:

1. Wash the cucumbers thoroughly under cold water. Dry them with a paper towel.
2. Cut the cucumbers into thin rounds with a sharp knife or a mandolin slicer. Spread the cucumber slices out on a serving tray or individual plates in a single layer.
3. In a small mixing dish, add low-fat cottage cheese, dill, chives, and lemon juice. Mix thoroughly until all components are uniformly distributed.
4. Season the cottage cheese mixture with salt and pepper, to taste. Adjust the seasoning to your liking.
5. Using a spoon, add a dollop of the cottage cheese mixture to each cucumber slice. For a more organised presentation, use a piping bag instead.
6. Once all of the cucumber slices have been covered with the cottage cheese mixture, sprinkle with fresh dill or chives to add colour and flavour.
7. Serve immediately as a refreshing snack or appetiser. Enjoy the sharpness of the cucumbers against the creamy richness of the cottage cheese.

Celery Sticks with Peanut Butter

Ingredients:

- 4 celery stalks, washed and trimmed
- ¼ cup natural peanut butter (no added sugar)

- Optional toppings: chopped nuts, chia seeds, or cinnamon (for added flavor)

Instructions:

1. **Prepare Celery Sticks:** carefully wash the celery stalks in cold water. Trim the stalks' ends and chop them into manageable sticks, each approximately 3-4 inches long.
2. **Spread Peanut Butter:** Using each celery stick, apply a small coating of natural peanut butter along the centre crease. Ensure that the peanut butter is uniformly distributed.
3. **Optional Toppings:** If preferred, top the peanut butter layer with chopped nuts, chia seeds, or a dash of cinnamon for more flavour and texture. These toppings not only improve the taste of the food, but also add to its nutritious content.
4. **Serve:** Place the prepared celery sticks and peanut butter on a serving plate or tray. To make the snack more enticing to seniors, arrange the sticks in a visually pleasing manner.
5. **Enjoy:** Serve celery sticks with peanut butter for a tasty and healthful snack. Encourage elders to appreciate the delightful crunch of celery and the creamy texture of peanut butter.

Hard-Boiled Eggs

Ingredients:

- 4 large eggs (or more, as desired)
- Water
- Ice cubes (optional, for ice bath)

Instructions:

1. Place the eggs in a saucepan in a single layer.
    Make sure the eggs aren't stacked on top of one
    another.
2. Pour enough cold water into the pot to cover the
    eggs by approximately an inch.
3. Place the pot over medium-high heat and come to
    a boil.
4. When the water has boiled, cover the saucepan
    with a lid and remove it from the heat. Allow the
    eggs to sit in the hot water for around 9-12
    minutes, depending on the desired level of
    doneness and egg size.
5. While the eggs fry, prepare a bowl of ice water.
    This will be used to swiftly chill the eggs once
    they are finished cooking.
6. After the eggs have boiled for the specified
    period of time, use a slotted spoon to transfer
    them to the bowl of icy water. Allow them to rest
    in the ice water bath for about 5 minutes to cool
    completely.
7. Once chilled, carefully tap the eggs on a hard
    surface to crack the shells, then peel them off
    with cold running water. This makes peeling
    easier.
8. Once peeled, hard-boiled eggs can be sliced and
    eaten as a snack, mixed into salads, or utilised in
    other recipes.

Caprese Skewers

Ingredients:
- 1 pint cherry tomatoes
- 8 ounces fresh mozzarella cheese, cut into cubes

- 1 bunch fresh basil leaves
- 2 tablespoons extra virgin olive oil
- 1 tablespoon balsamic vinegar (optional)
- Salt and pepper to taste
- Toothpicks or small skewers

Instructions:

1. **Prepare Ingredients:**
   - Rinse the cherry tomatoes and dry them with a paper towel.
   - Cut fresh mozzarella into bite-sized bits.
   - Wash and dry your fresh basil leaves.
2. **Assemble the Skewers:**
   - Thread one cherry tomato onto the bottom using a toothpick or small skewer.
   - Finish with a cube of fresh mozzarella cheese.
   - Finish by threading a fresh basil leaf onto a skewer.
   - Repeat until all of the ingredients are used.
3. **Arrange the Skewers:**
   - Arrange the prepared Caprese skewers on a serving plate.
4. **Drizzle with Olive Oil and Balsamic Vinegar:**
   - Drizzle extra virgin olive oil on the skewers.
   - You can also pour balsamic vinegar for extra flavour.
5. **Season with Salt and Pepper:**
   - Sprinkle salt and pepper to taste on the assembled skewers.
6. **Serve:**
   - Serve the Caprese skewers right away as an appetiser or as part of a light meal.

Edamame salad

Ingredients:
- 2 cups shelled edamame (frozen, thawed)
- 1 cup cherry tomatoes, halved
- 1/2 English cucumber, diced
- 1/4 cup red onion, finely chopped
- 2 tablespoons fresh cilantro, chopped
- 2 tablespoons fresh lime juice
- 1 tablespoon olive oil
- 1 garlic clove, minced
- Salt and pepper to taste

Instructions:
1. **Prepare the edamame:** Bring a pot of water to a boil before adding the shelled edamame. Boil for 3–5 minutes, or until tender. To halt the cooking process, drain and rinse well with cold water. Set aside.
2. **Mix the salad dressing** : In a small bowl, combine the fresh lime juice, olive oil, minced garlic, salt, and pepper. Adjust the seasoning to your taste.
3. **Combine Ingredients:** In a large mixing bowl, mix together the cooked edamame, halved cherry tomatoes, diced cucumber, finely chopped red onion, and fresh cilantro.
4. **Dress the salad:** Pour the prepared dressing over the salad mix. Gently toss the ingredients until uniformly coated with the dressing.
5. **Chill and Serve:** Cover the salad dish with plastic wrap or a cover and refrigerate for at least 30 minutes to allow the flavours to combine.

6. **Serve** : chilled as a delicious side dish or light supper. Before serving, you can add some more chopped cilantro as a garnish.

Greek Yogurt with Berries

Ingredients:
- 1/2 cup plain Greek yogurt (low-fat or non-fat for diabetes management)
- 1/2 cup mixed berries (such as strawberries, blueberries, raspberries)
- 1 tablespoon chopped nuts (almonds, walnuts, or pecans)
- 1 teaspoon honey or maple syrup (optional, for sweetness)
- 1/2 teaspoon ground cinnamon (optional, for addcd flavor)

Instructions:
1. **Prepare the Berries:**
   - Wash the berries thoroughly with cold water.
   - Dry them with a paper towel.
   - If using strawberries, hull and cut into bite-sized pieces.
2. **Assemble the Yogurt Bowl:**
   - In a serving bowl, spoon the Greek yoghurt.
3. **Add the Berries:**
   - Arrange the mixed berries on top of the yoghurt.
4. **Sprinkle with Nuts:**

- Sprinkle the chopped nuts over the berries. Nuts provide crunch and healthful fats to the dish.

5. **Drizzle with Honey or Maple Syrup (Optional):**
   - If desired, drizzle a small amount of honey or maple syrup over the yogurt and berries for added sweetness. Be mindful of the quantity, especially for diabetic diets.

6. **Sprinkle with Cinnamon (Optional):**
   - Sprinkle ground cinnamon over the yoghurt and berries to add more flavour. Cinnamon has the potential to help manage blood sugar levels.

7. **Serve:**
   - Serve immediately and enjoy this nutritious and pleasant Greek yoghurt with berries meal as a healthy snack or light breakfast.

Turkey and Cheese Roll-Ups

Ingredients:
- 8 slices of low-sodium turkey breast
- 4 slices of reduced-fat cheese (such as Swiss or cheddar)
- 1/2 cup of baby spinach leaves
- 1/4 cup of diced tomatoes (optional)
- 1/4 cup of diced bell peppers (optional)
- 1/4 cup of diced cucumbers (optional)
- 1/4 cup of light cream cheese, softened
- 1 tablespoon of Dijon mustard
- Salt and pepper to taste

Instructions:

1. Arrange the turkey slices on a clean surface. To eliminate any excess moisture, pat them dry with paper towels.
2. In a small mixing bowl, combine the softened cream cheese and Dijon mustard well. Season with salt and pepper to taste.
3. Spread a small coating of cream cheese mixture on each turkey slice.
4. Put a slice of cheese on top of the cream cheese mixture on each turkey slice.
5. Place a few baby spinach leaves on top of the cheese pieces. If desired, distribute the diced tomatoes, bell peppers, and cucumbers evenly among the spinach leaves.
6. Start at one end and tightly roll up each turkey slice with the filling ingredients inside.
7. Once folded up, fasten each roll using toothpicks to keep them together.
8. Using a sharp knife, gently cut each roll-up into bite-sized pieces about an inch thick.
9. Place the turkey and cheese roll-ups on a serving plate and serve immediately.

Roasted Vegetable Chips

Ingredients:

- 2 medium-sized carrots
- 2 medium-sized beets
- 1 medium-sized sweet potato
- 2 tablespoons olive oil
- 1/2 teaspoon salt

- 1/4 teaspoon black pepper
- 1/2 teaspoon garlic powder
- 1/2 teaspoon onion powder
- Cooking spray (optional)

Instructions:

1. **Preheat the oven:** to 375°F (190°C).
2. **Prepare the vegetables:** Wash and peel carrots, beets, and sweet potatoes. Thinly and uniformly slice the vegetables using a sharp knife or mandolin slicer. Thinner slices will yield crisper chips.
3. **Seasoning:** Toss the sliced veggies in olive oil in a large mixing basin until well coated. Then, season with salt, black pepper, garlic powder, and onion powder. Toss again until the seasoning is properly distributed on the veggies.
4. **Arrange on Baking Sheets** : Line baking pans with parchment paper or aluminium foil. Place the seasoned vegetable slices in a single layer on the baking sheets. Make sure they don't overlap to achieve even roasting.
5. **Roast the vegetables** : Place the baking sheets into the preheated oven Roast the vegetables for 25-30 minutes, or until they are crisp and faintly golden brown. Check the chips on occasion and flip the baking sheets as needed to ensure even cooking.
6. **Cool and Serve** : Once the vegetable chips are finished, take them from the oven and allow them to cool on the baking pans for a few minutes. This will allow them to get crispier. Move the chips to a serving plate or bowl.

7. **Optional Step** : If you want the vegetable slices to be extra crispy, simply coat them with cooking spray before seasoning. This will help them get crunchier while baking.
8. **Serve** : Roasted vegetable chips make a healthful snack. They can be eaten plain or with a low-sodium dip or hummus for extra flavour.

Avocado Salsa

Ingredients:
- 2 ripe avocados, diced
- 1 medium tomato, diced
- 1/4 cup red onion, finely chopped
- 1/4 cup fresh cilantro, chopped
- 1 jalapeño pepper, seeded and finely chopped (optional, adjust to taste)
- 1 clove garlic, minced
- Juice of 1 lime
- Salt and pepper to taste

Instructions:
1. In a medium mixing bowl, combine diced avocado, tomato, red onion, cilantro, jalapeño pepper (if using), and minced garlic.
2. Squeeze the juice from one lime over the avocado mixture. This not only provides flavour but also keeps the avocado from browning.
3. Gently toss all of the ingredients until completely combined. Make sure not to over-mash the avocado; some pieces are great for texture.
4. Season the avocado salsa with salt and pepper, to taste. Remember to begin with a tiny amount of salt and adjust as necessary.

5. Cover the bowl with plastic wrap or store the salsa in an airtight container. Refrigerate for at least 30 minutes to let the flavours to combine.
6. Before serving, give the salsa a brief swirl and taste to make any necessary flavour adjustments. If preferred, season with additional lime juice, salt, or pepper.
7. Avocado salsa can be served chilled as a dip with whole-grain chips or as a topping for grilled chicken or fish. Enjoy this refreshing and healthful treat!

Almond Stuffed Dates:

Ingredients:
- 12 large Medjool dates, pitted
- 12 whole almonds
- 1/4 teaspoon ground cinnamon (optional)
- 1/4 teaspoon vanilla extract (optional)

Instructions:
1. Preheat the oven to 350°F (175° C).
2. Using a small knife, carefully cut each date lengthwise, leaving a small opening. Be cautious not to cut all the way through; you want to make a pocket for the almond.
3. Insert one entire nut into each date, making sure it fits securely in the pocket.
4. If preferred, add a pinch of ground cinnamon to each date. You can also add a drop of vanilla extract to each date for added sweetness.
5. Place the packed dates on a baking sheet lined with parchment paper, leaving some space between each one.

6. Bake in a preheated oven for 8-10 minutes, or until the dates are slightly softened and the almonds are toasted.
7. Remove from the oven and allow it cool for a few minutes before serving.
8. Enjoy these delicious almond-stuffed dates as a sweet and filling snack!

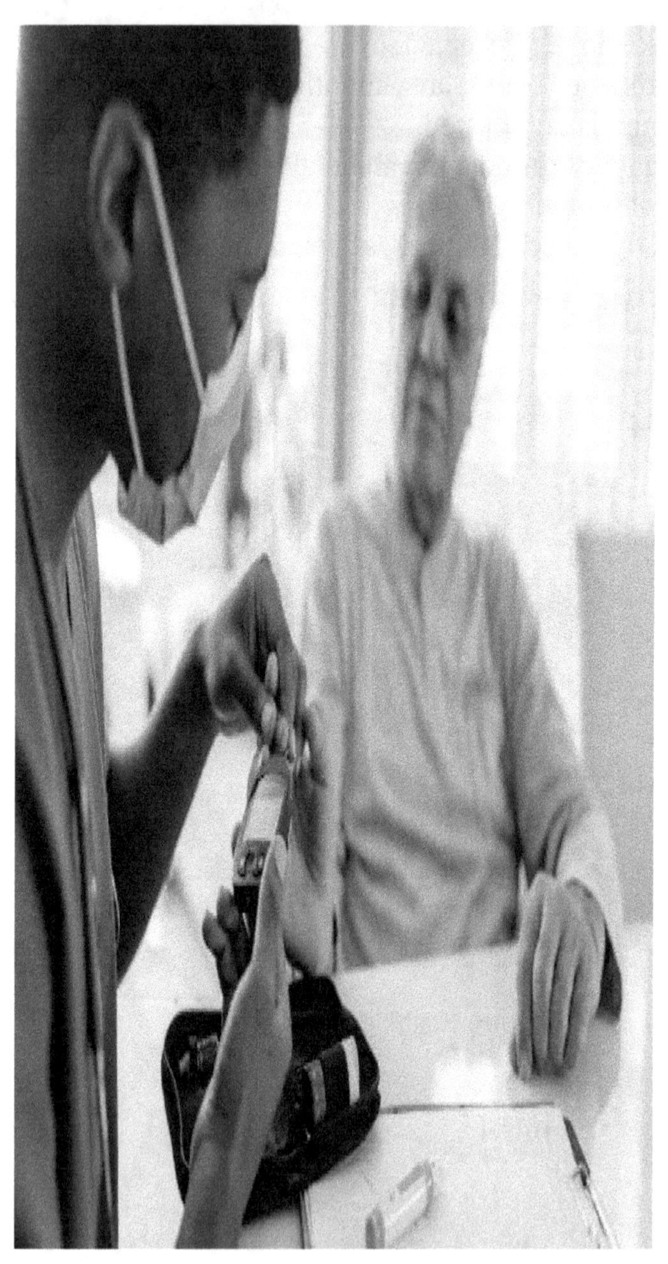

CHAPTER 6: BEVERAGES

Infused Water :

Ingredients:
- 1 medium cucumber, washed and sliced
- 1 lemon, washed and sliced
- 1 lime, washed and sliced
- 8-10 fresh mint leaves, washed
- 1.5 liters of water (filtered or spring water)

Instructions:
1. **Prepare the ingredients:** by properly washing the cucumber, lemon, and lime under cold running water. Cut them into thin circles or halves. Rinse your mint leaves as well.
2. **Combine Ingredients** : In a large pitcher, combine the sliced cucumber, lemon, lime, and mint leaves.
3. **Infuse Water** : Pour 1.5 litres of water into the pitcher, making sure to completely cover the cut ingredients.
4. **Refrigerate** : the pitcher for at least 2-4 hours, preferably overnight, to allow the flavours to combine.
5. **Serve Chilled:** If desired, serve the infused water over ice. Garnish each glass with a sprig of fresh mint for decoration.
6. **Storage** : Refrigerate the infused water for up to 2-3 days. After that, the flavours may begin to decrease.
7. **Variations** : Feel free to experiment with different fruits and herbs based on personal choice and availability. Some common varieties

include sliced strawberries, oranges, and even a few sprigs of rosemary.

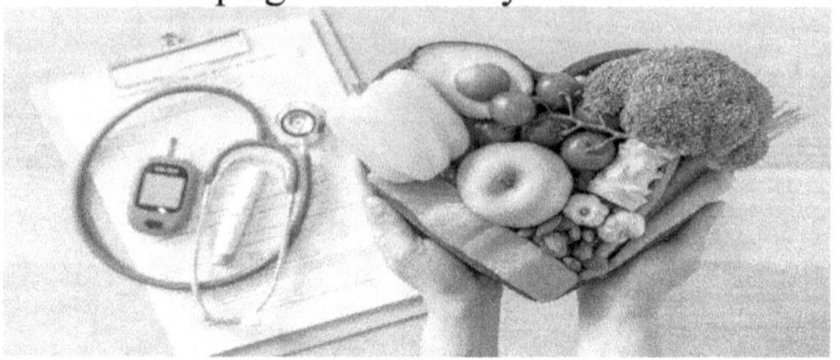

Herbal Tea

Ingredients:
- 2 teaspoons of dried hibiscus petals
- 1 teaspoon of dried chamomile flowers
- 1 teaspoon of dried cinnamon bark or 1 cinnamon stick
- 1 teaspoon of dried ginger root slices
- 4 cups of water
- Optional: Stevia or monk fruit sweetener to taste

Instructions:
1. **Prepare the Herbs:**
   - Gather your dried hibiscus petals, chamomile flowers, cinnamon bark or stick, and ginger root slices.
2. **Boil Water:**
   - Bring 4 cups of water to a boil in a medium pot over medium-high heat.
3. **Add Herbs:**
   - Once the water has reached a rolling boil, turn the heat down to low.

- Place the dried hibiscus petals, chamomile flowers, cinnamon bark or stick, and ginger root slices in the pot.

4. **Steep the Tea:**
   - Allow the herbs to steep in the hot water for about 10-15 minutes. This allows the flavours and beneficial compounds to infuse into the water.

5. **Strain the Tea:**
   - After steeping, take the pot from the heat.
   - To remove solid particles from the herbal tea, strain it through a fine mesh strainer or cheesecloth. You may discard the used herbs.

6. **Serve:**
   - Transfer the strained herbal tea to teacups or mugs.
   - If desired, add a little bit of stevia or monk fruit sweetener to taste. To keep the sugar content modest, limit the amount.

7. **Enjoy:**
   - Serve the herbal tea hot and savour the calming and comforting flavours.
   - Remember to keep portion sizes in check and speak with a healthcare practitioner before making nutritional choices, especially for seniors with diabetes.

Sparkling Water with Citrus

Ingredients:
- 1 liter of sparkling water
- 1 lemon

- 1 lime
- 1 orange
- Ice cubes (optional)
- Stevia or erythritol (optional, for sweetness)

Instructions:

1. **Prepare the Citrus Fruits:**
   - Wash the lemon, lime, and orange thoroughly with running water.
   - Cut the lemon, lime, and orange into thin rounds. Remove any seeds.
2. **Chill the Sparkling Water:**
   - Place the litre of sparkling water in the refrigerator for at least 1 hour before preparing the drink. Chilled sparkling water ensures a refreshing taste.
3. **Assemble the Drink:**
   - Grab a large pitcher or serving jug.
   - If you want it extra cold, add some ice cubes to the pitcher.
4. **Add Citrus Slices:**
   - Carefully add the sliced lemon, lime, and orange rounds to the pitcher.
5. **Pour in Sparkling Water:** Once the water has been sufficiently cold, carefully pour it into the pitcher with the citrus pieces.
6. **Optional: Add Sweetener:**
   - If desired, sweeten the sparkling citrus water with a few drops liquid stevia or a teaspoon erythritol. Stir gently until dissolved.
7. **Mix Gently:**
   - Using a long spoon or a stirrer, gently combine the ingredients. To keep the

sparkling water's sparkle, don't shake it too vigorously.

8. **Serve:**
   - Pour the sparkling citrus water into separate glasses or serving cups.
   - Garnish each glass with a fresh slice of lemon, lime, or orange for added decoration.
9. **Enjoy:**
   - Serve the delightful sparkling citrus water immediately.
   - Sip and savour the zesty flavours while staying hydrated all day.

Green Smoothies

Ingredients:
- 2 cups fresh spinach leaves, thoroughly washed
- 1 ripe avocado, peeled and pitted
- 1 medium cucumber, peeled and chopped
- 1 small Granny Smith apple, cored and chopped
- 1/2 cup unsweetened almond milk (or any unsweetened plant-based milk)
- 1 tablespoon fresh lemon juice
- 1 teaspoon ground cinnamon (optional)
- Ice cubes (optional, for a colder smoothie)

Instructions:
1. **Prepare the ingredients:** by carefully washing the spinach leaves and chopping the cucumber and apple into small parts for better blending.
2. **Ingredients:** In a blender, combine spinach leaves, avocado, diced cucumber, chopped apple,

almond milk, fresh lemon juice, and ground cinnamon (if using).

3. **Blend:** Combine all of the ingredients until smooth. If the recipe is too thick, add a little more almond milk until you get the ideal consistency.
4. **Taste and Adjust:** Adjust the sweetness or sharpness of the smoothie by adding extra lemon juice as needed.
5. **Serve:** Pour the green smoothie into glasses. If you like, add a few ice cubes to each glass to chill the smoothie.
6. **Enjoy:** Serve the green smoothies immediately to appreciate their refreshing flavour and nutritional value.

Iced Coffee with Unsweetened Almond Milk

Ingredients:
- 1 cup brewed coffee, chilled
- 1/2 cup unsweetened almond milk
- Ice cubes
- Optional: sugar-free sweetener or sugar substitute (as per individual preference)
- Optional: whipped cream for topping (sugar-free if preferred)

Instructions:
1. **Brew Coffee** : Begin by making your preferred coffee blend. If you want a more intense flavour, make it stronger.
2. **Chill Coffee** : Let the brewed coffee cool to room temperature. To speed up the procedure,

refrigerate it for about 30 minutes or pour it over ice.

3. **Prepare almond milk:** Measure out 1/2 cup of unsweetened almond milk. You can use store-bought almond milk or make your own if desired.
4. **Sweeten (optional):** Add your favourite sugar-free sweetener or sugar replacement to the iced coffee. Stir well until the sweetness is completely dissolved.
5. **Combine Ingredients:** Fill a tumbler with ice cubes. Pour the chilled coffee over the ice, leaving enough space at the top of the glass.
6. **Add almond milk:** Pour unsweetened almond milk over the coffee and ice.
7. **Stir** : Using a spoon or stir stick, carefully combine the coffee and almond milk.
8. **Optional Toppings:** If preferred, top your iced coffee with whipped cream. If you're trying to limit your sugar intake, use sugar-free whipped cream.
9. **Serve:** Your delightful Iced Coffee with Unsweetened Almond Milk is ready to drink! Stir again before serving to ensure that all of the flavours are completely blended.

Coconut Water

Ingredients:
- 1 cup fresh coconut water
- Ice cubes (optional)
- Fresh lime or lemon wedges for garnish (optional)
- Mint leaves for garnish (optional)

Instructions:
1. **Selecting the Coconut:**
   - Choose a fresh, young coconut that is free of cracks and mould. When you gently shake the container, you should hear water sloshing inside.
2. **Opening the Coconut:**
   - Put the coconut on a stable surface. Use a hefty knife or cleaver to carefully cut off the top, leaving a small opening to access the water.
3. **Collecting the Water:**
   - Tilt the coconut over a clean glass or basin to let the water escape. To eliminate particles, strain the water over a fine mesh sieve.
4. **Chilling the Coconut Water:**
   - Place the strained coconut water in the refrigerator for about 30 minutes, or until it reaches the appropriate temperature.
5. **Serving:**
   - Pour the chilled coconut water into a glass with ice cubes, if preferred.
   - Squeeze a wedge of fresh lime or lemon into the coconut water for a citrusy twist.
   - Garnish with a sprig of mint leaves for a refreshing aroma and flavour.
6. **Enjoy :**
   - Stir the coconut water gently to mix in the flavours.
   - Sip and enjoy this hydrating and nutritious beverage as part of your diabetes-friendly diet.

Vegetable Juice

Ingredients:
- 2 medium-sized carrots, peeled and chopped
- 2 stalks of celery, chopped
- 1 medium-sized beetroot, peeled and chopped
- 1 large cucumber, peeled and chopped
- 2 cups spinach leaves, washed
- 1 green apple, cored and chopped
- 1-inch piece of ginger, peeled
- 1 lemon, juiced
- 2 cups water
- Ice cubes (optional)

Instructions:
1. Wash and prepare all of the vegetables and fruits. Make sure they're completely washed and peeled if required.
2. To make it easier to juice, chop the carrots, celery, beetroot, cucumber, and green apple into small pieces.
3. Peel the ginger and cut it into tiny slices to improve the flavour of the juice.
4. In a high-speed blender or juicer, combine the carrots, celery, beetroot, cucumber, spinach leaves, green apple, and ginger.
5. Squeeze the juice of one lemon into a blender or juicer. The lemon imparts a tart flavour that balances the sweetness of the vegetables and fruits.
6. Add 2 cups of water to the blender to help with the juicing process and to change the consistency of the juice.

7. Blend all of the ingredients until smooth and properly incorporated. If using a juicer, follow the manufacturer's juicing instructions.
8. Once the juice is ready, taste it and adjust the flavour as needed. You can add more lemon juice for sharpness or a green apple for sweetness, depending on your taste.
9. If desired, add ice cubes to the juice to make it more refreshing, particularly in hot weather.
10. Pour the veggie juice into glasses and serve immediately. Consume the nutritious and diabetic-friendly beverage as a refreshing snack or as part of a meal.

Homemade Lemonade

Ingredients:
- 4 large lemons, juiced (about 1 cup of fresh lemon juice)
- 4 cups of cold water
- 1/4 cup of granulated sugar substitute (such as stevia or erythritol)
- Ice cubes (optional)
- Lemon slices or mint sprigs for garnish (optional)

Instructions:
1. Begin by juicing lemons. Roll each lemon on the counter to release the juice before chopping and juicing. You should aim for approximately 1 cup of fresh lemon juice.
2. In a pitcher, combine freshly squeezed lemon juice and 4 cups cold water. Stir well to ensure that the lemon juice and water are properly distributed.

3. Gradually add the granulated sugar alternative to the lemon water mixture, stirring constantly until dissolved entirely. Adjust the sweetness to your taste. Remember that a diabetic-friendly recipe should have a minimal sugar content.

4. When the sugar substitute has completely dissolved, taste the lemonade and adjust the sweetness or sharpness as needed by adding additional lemon juice or sugar substitute.

5. If desired, add ice cubes to the pitcher to chill the lemonade even further. To enhance the flavour and completely chill the lemonade, refrigerate it for at least 30 minutes before serving.

6. Serve the diabetic-friendly homemade lemonade in glasses with ice cubes. Garnish each glass with a slice of lemon or a sprig of fresh mint for added freshness and visual appeal.

7. To ensure equitable distribution of sweetness, stir the lemonade before pouring it into glasses. Enjoy your delightful, diabetic-friendly homemade lemonade!

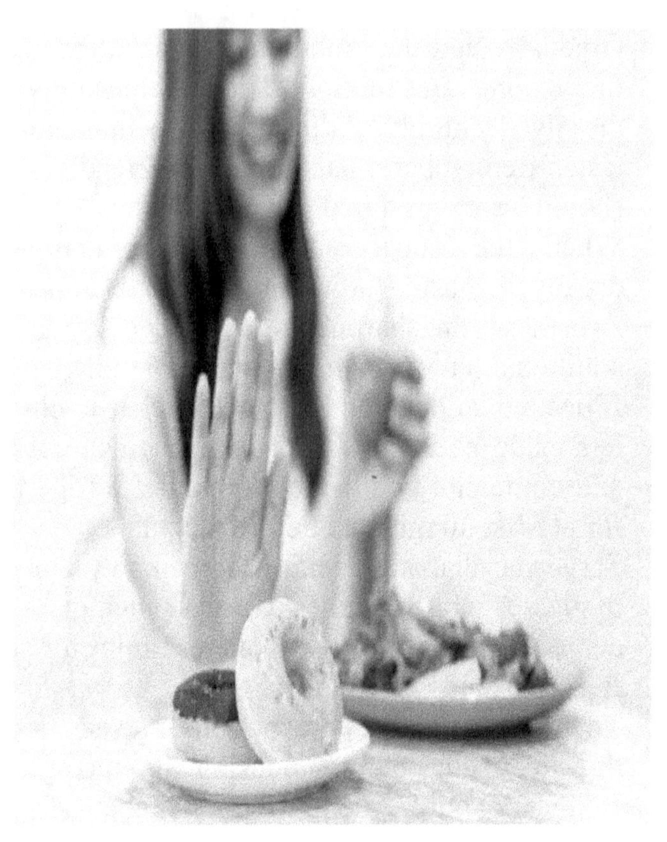

CONCLUSION

Additional resources

A comprehensive diabetes diet cookbook for seniors should include a variety of supplementary tools to help them maintain their health and well-being. These resources include a wide range of issues, including nutritional information and meal planning recommendations, as well as lifestyle management techniques and advice on dealing with the challenges of diabetes. Here are some important websites that might substantially aid seniors with diabetes:

1. **Nutritional supervision:** Seniors with diabetes frequently require individualised nutritional supervision. The cookbook should include thorough information on carbohydrate counting, portion control, and glycemic index management to assist seniors in making informed dietary decisions. Teaching elders how to read nutrition labels and understand dietary requirements can help them take control of their nutrition.

2. **Meal Planning Tools:** A diabetes diet cookbook should include useful meal planning tools including sample meal plans, grocery shopping lists, and meal preparation advice. These tools can assist seniors in planning healthy meals that meet their nutritional needs while properly managing blood sugar levels. Encouraging variety and moderation in food choices can make meal preparation more fun and sustainable for seniors.

3. **Healthy Cooking Techniques:** Seniors may benefit from learning about healthy cooking methods that can improve the nutritional value of their meals while lowering fat, sodium, and sugar. The cookbook should include instructions for baking, grilling, steaming, and sautéing to produce delicious and nutritious meals without sacrificing taste or texture.

4. **Ingredient Substitutions:** Many classic dishes can be made diabetic-friendly by substituting ingredients with lower carbohydrate and sugar content. The cookbook should offer a list of

product substitutions and alternative sweeteners that seniors can utilise to change up their favourite recipes while still eating flavorful and satisfying meals.

5. **Tips for Dining Out:** Eating out can be difficult for seniors with diabetes since restaurant meals frequently contain hidden sugars, harmful fats, and big portions. The cookbook should include practical dining ideas and tactics, such as pre-planning menus, selecting restaurants with healthier selections, and exercising portion control when eating out.

6. **Physical activity recommendations:** Regular physical exercise is a vital component of diabetes therapy, helping to improve insulin sensitivity, control blood sugar levels, and maintain overall health and mobility. The cookbook should include recommendations for incorporating physical activity into daily routines, such as walking, swimming, yoga, or chair exercises tailored to seniors' needs and abilities.

7. **Monitoring and Self-Care:** Seniors with diabetes should be encouraged to monitor their blood sugar levels regularly and stay vigilant for signs of hypo- or hyperglycemia. The cookbook can provide guidance on self-care practices, including medication management, stress reduction techniques, and seeking medical support when needed. Emphasizing the importance of regular check-ups with healthcare providers can help seniors stay proactive about managing their diabetes effectively.

8. **Community Support and Resources:** Living with diabetes can be challenging, but seniors don't have to face it alone. The cookbook should emphasise the value of getting help from friends, family, support groups, and diabetes educators. Providing information about local services, online forums, and instructional programmes can help seniors connect with essential support networks and handle their diabetes journey confidently.

By combining these additional resources into a diabetes diet cookbook for seniors, carers and healthcare professionals can help older persons make good lifestyle choices, properly manage their diabetes, and live a fulfilling and active life. Seniors can adopt a diabetes-friendly diet that improves long-term health and well-being with knowledge, support, and practical direction .

www.ingramcontent.com/pod-product-compliance
Lightning Source LLC
Chambersburg PA
CBHW050843260726
48660CB00006B/2406